NATURAL HAIR CARE RECIPES

A wholesome alternative
homemade shampoo, conditioner
and treatments to promote scalp
health and prevent hair loss.

Shane Ramiro

Table of Contents

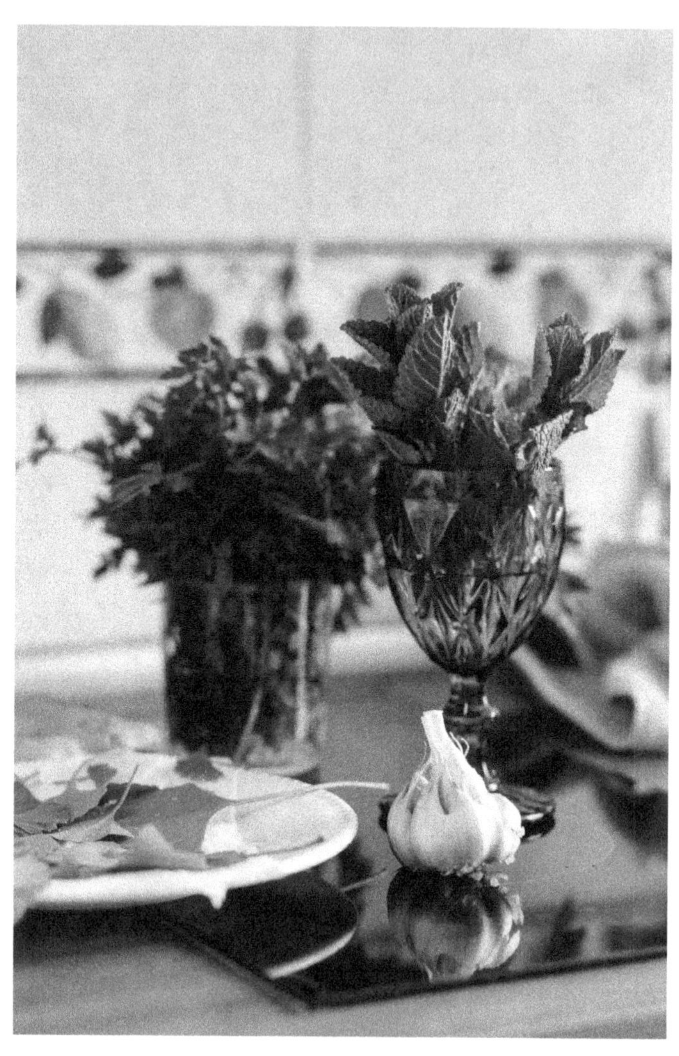

Introduction

In a world buzzing with synthetic solutions, there's a quiet resurgence of reverence for nature's wisdom—especially when it comes to hair care. Amidst the shelves of commercial products laden with chemicals, natural hair care recipes emerge as beacons of authenticity and well-being. This is a journey back to basics, where the lush offerings of the earth hold the key to luscious, vibrant locks.

Our story begins with the realization that the simplicity of natural ingredients can be profound. From the soothing embrace of aloe vera to the nourishing richness of coconut oil, the world of natural hair care is a treasure trove waiting to be explored. Each ingredient carries not just the promise of healthier hair but also a connection to the earth's bounty.

Picture a kitchen transformed into an alchemist's den, where herbs and oils are blended with care. These recipes aren't just concoctions; they're rituals, a celebration of the symbiotic relationship between nature and our hair. The allure lies not only in the effectiveness of these recipes but also in the mindful process of crafting them.

As we embark on this journey, we'll uncover the secrets of hibiscus-infused rinses, the magic of avocado masks, and the simplicity of rosemary-scented oils. Natural hair care isn't a trend; it's a return to the roots, an ode to the age-old wisdom that whispers through the leaves and petals. So, let's dive into the world of natural hair care recipes—a harmonious blend of tradition, nature, and the vibrant essence of self-care.

Chapter one

Natural hair care recipes

Natural hair care recipes embrace the philosophy that the healthiest solutions for our hair are often rooted in nature's bounty. By relying on plant-based ingredients and avoiding harsh chemicals, these recipes cater to a growing desire for holistic and sustainable hair care practices. Let's explore the comprehensive world of natural hair care recipes, understanding the ingredients, methods, and benefits that make them increasingly popular.

Ingredients:

1. Aloe Vera:

Known for its soothing properties, aloe vera is a staple in natural hair care. Its gel hydrates the scalp, promotes hair growth, and adds a natural sheen.

2. Coconut Oil:

A versatile elixir, coconut oil deeply nourishes hair, prevents protein loss, and can be used for oil massages or as a pre-shampoo treatment.

3. Avocado:

Rich in vitamins and healthy fats, avocados make excellent hair masks. They moisturize, add shine, and strengthen hair strands.

4. Hibiscus:

Hibiscus flowers are cherished for their ability to stimulate hair growth, combat dandruff, and enhance the natural color of hair.

5. Rosemary:

Rosemary-infused oil promotes scalp health, strengthens hair, and may prevent premature graying.

Methods:

1. DIY Hair Masks:

Blend ingredients like mashed avocado, honey, and coconut oil to create nourishing masks that can be applied to damp hair, left on for 20-30 minutes, and then rinsed.

2. Herbal Rinses:

Prepare herbal infusions using hibiscus, chamomile, or rosemary. These rinses can be used after shampooing to add shine, balance pH, and promote scalp health.

3. Oil Treatments:

Apply warm coconut oil or a mix of oils like jojoba and argan to the scalp and hair, leaving it on for an hour or overnight. This helps with deep conditioning and repairing damaged strands.

Benefits:

Chemical-Free:

1. Natural recipes eliminate exposure to harsh chemicals commonly found in commercial products, reducing the risk of irritation and damage.

Promotes Scalp Health:

2. Ingredients like aloe vera, hibiscus, and rosemary have antimicrobial properties that foster a healthy scalp environment.

Sustainability:

3. Many natural ingredients are eco-friendly and sustainable, aligning with the principles of conscious living.

Customizable:

4. Individuals can tailor recipes to their specific hair needs, whether it's moisture retention, volume, or addressing specific concerns like dandruff.

Cost-Effective:

5. Creating homemade hair care products
    can often be more budget-friendly than
    purchasing high-end commercial
    alternatives.

Natural hair care recipes embody a return to
simplicity, a celebration of the Earth's gifts, and
a commitment to healthier, more sustainable
living. As individuals seek a deeper connection
with their hair and the environment, these
recipes offer a personalized and mindful
approach to nurturing one's tresses.

Natural hair care homemade recipes

1. Coconut Oil and Honey Mask:

- **Ingredients:**
    - 3 tablespoons coconut oil
    - 2 tablespoons honey
- **Method:**
    - Blend the honey and coconut oil until well blended.
    - Make sure the mixture covers all of the moist hair.
    - Leave on for 30–60 minutes before washing with a gentle shampoo.

This mask deeply nourishes and moisturizes, leaving hair silky and manageable.

2. Aloe Vera and Olive Oil Treatment:

- **Ingredients:**
    - 1/4 cup aloe vera gel
    - 2 tablespoons olive oil
- **Method:**
    - Blend aloe vera gel and olive oil until smooth.
    - Apply the mixture to the hair, focusing on the roots and tips.
    - After letting it rest for 20 to 30 minutes, give it a good rinse.

This treatment promotes scalp health and adds a natural shine to your hair.

3. Avocado and Banana Hair Mask:

- **Ingredients:**
  - 1 ripe avocado
  - 1 ripe banana
- **Method:**
  - Banana and avocado should be mashed into a smooth paste.
  - After dampening your hair and applying the mixture, put on a shower hat.
  - Rinse after 30–45 minutes and shampoo as usual.

Packed with vitamins and healthy fats, this mask strengthens and revitalizes dull hair.

4. Rosemary Infused Vinegar Rinse:

- **Ingredients:**

- o   2 tablespoons dried rosemary

  - o   1 cup apple cider vinegar

- **Method:**

  - o   Infuse dried rosemary in apple cider vinegar for one week.

  - o   Dilute the infused vinegar with water (1:1 ratio) and use it as a final hair rinse after shampooing.

Rosemary promotes scalp health and adds a lustrous shine to your hair.

5. Hibiscus and Fenugreek Hair Paste:

- **Ingredients:**

  - o   Handful of dried hibiscus petals

  - o   2 tablespoons fenugreek seeds

- **Method:**

- Soak hibiscus petals and fenugreek seeds in water overnight.
- Blend into a paste and apply to the hair, focusing on the scalp.
- Leave for 30 minutes before washing thoroughly.

This paste stimulates hair growth and helps manage frizz.

Consistency is Key:

- Regular use of these homemade recipes yields better results over time.

Adjust to Your Hair Type:

- Modify ingredient proportions based on your hair's needs, whether it's dry, oily, or normal.

Use Quality Ingredients:

- Opt for organic and pure ingredients to maximize the benefits for your hair.

Embrace the natural goodness of these homemade recipes for a healthier, more vibrant mane. Experiment with ingredients to discover the perfect concoction tailored to your unique hair care needs.

Chapter two

How to make incredible shampoo

Creating an incredible homemade shampoo allows you to control the ingredients, ensuring a natural and customized blend tailored to your hair's specific needs. Here's a simple recipe to make a nourishing and revitalizing shampoo:

DIY Nourishing Shampoo Recipe:

Ingredients:

1. **Liquid Castile Soap (1/2 cup):**
   - Acts as the base for cleansing without stripping natural oils.

2. **Coconut Milk (1/4 cup):**
   - Adds moisture and nourishment to the hair.

3. **Jojoba Oil (1 tablespoon):**

- Helps balance the scalp's natural oils without causing greasiness.

4. **Aloe Vera Gel (2 tablespoons):**

   - Soothes the scalp, promotes hair growth, and adds a silky texture.

5. **Essential Oils (10-15 drops):**

   - Choose oils like lavender, tea tree, or peppermint for their therapeutic properties and pleasant fragrance.

Instructions:

1. **Mixing the Base:**

   - In a bowl, combine the liquid castile soap, coconut milk, jojoba oil, and aloe vera gel. To achieve an equal mix, thoroughly stir.

2. **Adding Essential Oils:**

- Incorporate your chosen essential oils, adjusting the quantity based on your preference. Essential oils not only enhance the scent but also contribute to the overall health of your hair and scalp.

3. **Blending:**
   - To get a smooth consistency, mix using an immersion blender or blender. This step helps combine the ingredients thoroughly, ensuring a uniform shampoo texture.

4. **Storage:**
   - Transfer the mixture into a clean, empty shampoo bottle or container. A funnel can be helpful for this step.

5. **Usage:**

   ○ Shake the bottle before each use. Apply a small amount to wet hair, lather, and massage into the scalp. Rinse thoroughly with water.

Tips for an Incredible Shampoo:

1. **pH Balance:**

   ○ Adjust the recipe to achieve a balanced pH, ensuring it aligns with the natural pH of your hair.

2. **Hair Type Consideration:**

   ○ Customize the shampoo based on your hair type. For example, add more coconut milk for extra moisture or adjust essential oils for specific benefits.

3. **Experiment Gradually:**

- Introduce one new ingredient at a time and observe how your hair responds. This way, you can identify which components work best for you.

4. **Consistency is Key:**

    - Give your hair time to adjust to the natural shampoo. It may take a few washes before you notice the full benefits.

By crafting your own shampoo, you not only enjoy a personalized hair care experience but also contribute to a more sustainable and eco-friendly approach to beauty. Explore variations and find the perfect blend that leaves your hair feeling refreshed, healthy, and incredible.

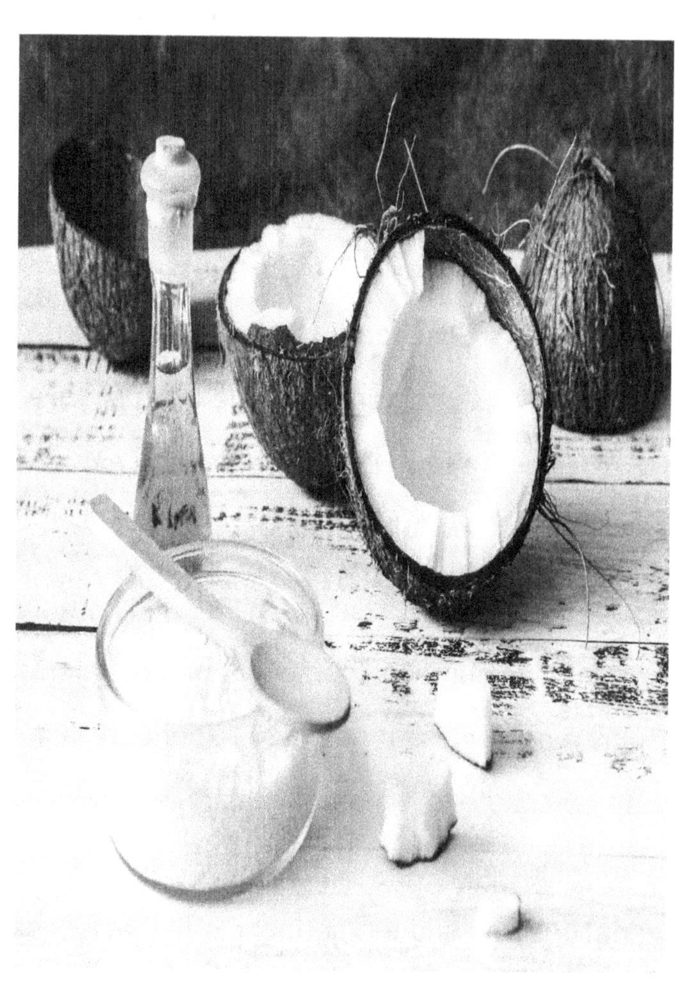

Chapter three

Apple Cider Vinegar

Apple Cider Vinegar: A Versatile Elixir for Health and Beauty

Introduction:

Crushed apples are fermented to create apple cider vinegar (ACV). Beyond its culinary uses, ACV has gained popularity for its diverse benefits in health and beauty. Packed with enzymes, probiotics, and beneficial acids, this amber-hued elixir has become a staple in natural wellness routines.

Health Benefits:

1. Digestive Aid:
    - ACV may aid digestion by promoting the production of

stomach acid, helping alleviate indigestion and bloating.

2. Blood Sugar Regulation:

    o   Some studies suggest that ACV may help stabilize blood sugar levels, making it a potential ally for individuals managing diabetes.

3. Weight Management:

    o   Including ACV in your diet may contribute to feelings of fullness, potentially supporting weight loss efforts.

4. Heart Health:

    o   The acetic acid in ACV may help lower cholesterol levels and improve heart health.

Beauty and Hair Care:

1. **Balancing pH:**

   - ACV has a pH level close to that of human hair, making it an excellent natural conditioner that helps balance the scalp's pH.

2. **Clarifying Hair Rinse:**

   - A diluted ACV rinse can remove product buildup, clarify the hair, and add shine. Use one part apple cider vinegar to two parts water as a last rinse after shampooing.

3. **Skin Toner:**

   - Diluted ACV can act as a natural toner, helping to balance the skin's pH and reduce acne.

4. **Sunburn Relief:**

- A mixture of ACV and water can soothe sunburned skin, providing relief and aiding in the healing process.

Incorporating ACV Into Your Routine:

1. **Internal Consumption:**

   - Mix 1-2 tablespoons of ACV in a glass of water and drink before meals. Adding honey or a splash of lemon can enhance the taste.

2. **Hair Rinse:**

   - After shampooing, pour the diluted ACV rinse over your hair, allowing it to sit for a few minutes before rinsing with water.

3. **Facial Toner:**

- Mix one part ACV with two parts water and apply to the face using a cotton pad as a natural toner.

4. **Bath Soak:**

   - Add a cup of ACV to your bathwater for a relaxing soak that may benefit your skin.

Caution and Considerations:

Dilution is Key:

- Always dilute ACV before use, especially on the skin or hair, to prevent irritation.

Consultation:

- Individuals with specific health conditions or concerns should consult a healthcare professional before incorporating ACV into their routine.

Apple cider vinegar's versatility extends beyond the kitchen, making it a valuable addition to holistic health and beauty practices. Whether sipped in a morning drink or applied as a natural tonic for hair and skin, this humble elixir continues to inspire a range of wellness benefits.

Chapter four

Essential Oils

Essential Oils: Nature's Aromatic Essence for Health and Well-being

Introduction:

Essential oils are concentrated plant extracts that capture the aromatic essence, flavor, and therapeutic properties of various botanicals. These volatile oils have been used for centuries across diverse cultures, offering a myriad of benefits for physical, mental, and emotional well-being.

Extraction Process:

Different techniques, including as solvent extraction, steam distillation, and cold pressing, are used to extract essential oils. This meticulous process ensures the preservation of the plant's active compounds, resulting in potent and fragrant oils.

Common Essential Oils and Their Benefits:

1. Lavender Oil:
    - Calming and versatile, lavender oil promotes relaxation, aids in sleep, and soothes skin irritations.

2. Peppermint Oil:
    - Invigorating and refreshing, peppermint oil can alleviate headaches, boost energy, and aid digestion.

3. Tea Tree Oil:
    - Recognized for its antibacterial and antifungal properties, tea tree oil is often used to treat skin

conditions and promote a healthy
scalp.

4. Eucalyptus Oil:

   o Known for its respiratory benefits,
     eucalyptus oil can ease
     congestion and promote clear
     breathing.

5. Lemon Oil:

   o Uplifting and cleansing, lemon oil
     is used to enhance mood,
     support digestion, and even as a
     natural cleaner.

Applications and Usage:

1. Aromatherapy:

   o Diffusing essential oils in the air
     can create a calming or
     invigorating atmosphere,
     influencing mood and emotions.

2. Topical Application:

   - Diluted with a carrier oil, essential oils can be applied to the skin for massage, skincare, or targeted relief.

3. Inhalation:

   - Inhaling the aroma of essential oils can have immediate effects on the respiratory system and emotional state.

4. Bath Soaks:

   - Adding a few drops of essential oils to a bath creates a relaxing and aromatic experience.

Safety Considerations:

1. Dilution:

   - Essential oils are potent and should be diluted before direct

skin application. A common ratio
is 1–2 drops per teaspoon of
carrier oil.

2. Patch Test:

    ○ Always perform a patch test
       before applying a new essential
       oil to the skin to check for any
       adverse reactions.

3. Pregnancy and Medical Conditions:

    ○ Pregnant individuals or those with
       specific health conditions should
       consult a healthcare professional
       before using certain essential
       oils.

Conclusion:

Essential oils offer a holistic approach to
well-being, combining the power of nature with
sensory pleasures. Whether used for

relaxation, skincare, or aromatherapy, these aromatic extracts have woven themselves into rituals that promote balance and harmony in our lives. As with any natural remedy, understanding their properties and proper usage ensures a safe and enjoyable experience with essential oils.

Chapter five

Coconut oils

Coconut Oil: Nature's Versatile Elixir for Health and Beauty

Introduction:

Coconut oil, extracted from the meat of coconuts, has long been revered for its diverse applications in health, beauty, and culinary pursuits. With a unique combination of fatty acids, vitamins, and antioxidants, coconut oil has earned a well-deserved reputation as a versatile and nourishing elixir.

Nutrient Profile:

1. Medium-Chain Fatty Acids (MCFAs):
   - The predominant fatty acids in coconut oil, such as lauric acid,

provide a quick and efficient
source of energy for the body.

2. Vitamins and Antioxidants:

   ○ Coconut oil contains vitamin E,
     which contributes to skin health,
     and antioxidants that help combat
     oxidative stress.

Health Benefits:

1. Heart Health:

   ○ MCFAs in coconut oil may
     contribute to heart health by
     raising levels of good cholesterol
     (HDL) and promoting a healthy
     lipid profile.

2. Brain Function:

   ○ The ketones produced from
     MCFAs are believed to provide
     an alternative energy source for

the brain, potentially aiding

cognitive function.

3. Immune Support:

    ○   Lauric acid, abundant in coconut

        oil, exhibits antimicrobial and

        antiviral properties that may

        support the immune system.

Beauty and Skincare:

1. Moisturizing Agent:

    ○   Coconut oil's natural emollient

        properties make it an effective

        moisturizer for skin and hair.

2. Makeup Remover:

    ○   Its ability to dissolve makeup and

        impurities makes coconut oil an

        excellent and gentle makeup

        remover.

3. Hair Care:

- Applying coconut oil as a hair mask can enhance shine, reduce frizz, and contribute to overall hair health.

Culinary Uses:

1. Cooking and Baking:
   - Coconut oil's high smoke point makes it suitable for various cooking methods, and its pleasant flavor complements both savory and sweet dishes.
2. Coffee or Tea Boost:
   - Some individuals incorporate coconut oil into their coffee or tea as a source of sustained energy.

Tips for Usage:

1. Virgin vs. Refined:

- Choose virgin, unrefined coconut oil for a more pronounced coconut flavor and a higher nutrient content.

2. Skin Patch Test:

   - Before applying to a larger area, perform a patch test when using coconut oil on the skin to ensure there are no adverse reactions.

3. Incorporate Into Diet Gradually:

   - If using coconut oil for dietary purposes, introduce it gradually to avoid potential digestive discomfort.

Conclusion:

Coconut oil, with its multitude of applications, stands as a testament to the richness of nature's offerings. Whether used for nourishing the body from within, enhancing beauty routines, or elevating culinary creations, coconut oil continues to be a staple that transcends cultural boundaries. Embracing the holistic benefits of this tropical elixir adds a touch of nature's goodness to our daily lives.

Emu oils

Emu Oil: Nature's Soothing Elixir for Skin and Hair

Introduction:

Derived from the fat of the emu bird native to Australia, emu oil has gained popularity for its therapeutic properties. Rich in essential fatty acids and other bioactive compounds, this natural oil is renowned for its potential benefits in skincare and hair care.

Nutrient Composition:

1. Omega Fatty Acids:
   - Emu oil is a source of omega-3, omega-6, and omega-9 fatty acids, which are crucial for maintaining skin health.
2. Vitamins:
   - It contains vitamins A and E, known for their antioxidant properties that contribute to skin rejuvenation.
3. Anti-Inflammatory Compounds:
   - Bioactive compounds in emu oil, such as oleic acid and linoleic acid, exhibit anti-inflammatory effects.

Skincare Benefits:

1. Moisturization:

    o   Emu oil's ability to deeply
        penetrate the skin provides
        intense hydration, making it a
        potent moisturizer.

2. Anti-Aging Properties:

    o   The antioxidants in emu oil may
        assist in reducing the appearance
        of fine lines and wrinkles,
        promoting a more youthful
        complexion.

3. Wound Healing:

    o   Emu oil's anti-inflammatory and
        skin-nourishing properties may
        aid in wound healing and scar
        reduction.

Hair Care:

1. Scalp Health:

    o Massaging emu oil into the scalp
      can help alleviate dryness,
      reduce dandruff, and promote
      overall scalp health.

2. Hair Moisture:

    o Applying emu oil to the hair can
      add moisture, improve texture,
      and reduce frizz.

Joint and Muscle Relief:

1. Anti-Inflammatory Effects:

    o Emu oil's anti-inflammatory
      properties make it a popular
      choice for soothing joint and
      muscle discomfort.

2. Arthritis Support:

- Some individuals use emu oil topically for arthritis, finding relief from pain and inflammation.

Usage Tips:

1. Patch Test:
   - Before applying emu oil widely, perform a patch test to ensure there are no adverse reactions, especially for those with sensitive skin.

2. Choose Pure and High-Quality Oils:
   - Opt for pure, undiluted emu oil from reputable sources to ensure its effectiveness.

3. Storage:
   - Store emu oil in a cool, dark place to prevent oxidation and maintain its potency.

Conclusion:

Emu oil, with its array of beneficial compounds, stands as a natural remedy for skin and hair care. While individual experiences may vary, many users find comfort and relief in incorporating this soothing elixir into their beauty and wellness routines. As with any natural product, understanding its properties and proper usage enhances the potential benefits it can offer.

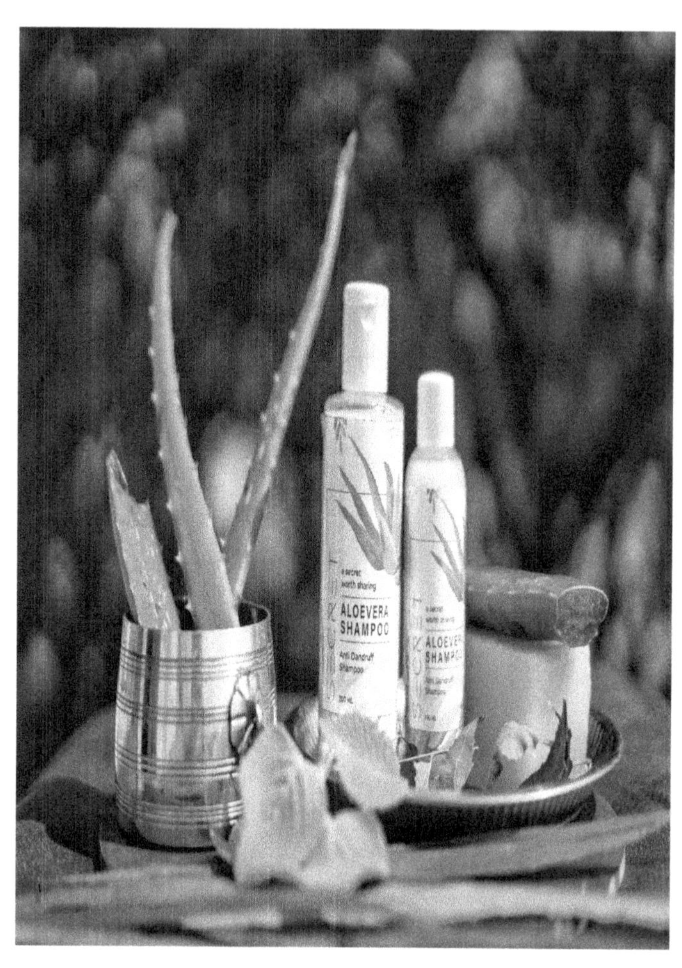

a secret
worth sharing
ALOEVERA
SHAMPOO
Anti Dandruff
Shampoo
ALOEVERA
SHAMPOO

Chapter six

Favorite foaming shampoo

Embracing the Blissful Bubbles: A Dive into My Favorite Foaming Shampoo

Introduction:

In the bustling world of hair care, finding a favorite foaming shampoo can be a transformative experience. The sensory pleasure of rich, velvety lather coupled with effective cleansing is a ritual that turns a mundane task into a moment of indulgence.

The Chosen Foaming Shampoo:

My go-to foaming shampoo boasts a perfect blend of cleansing power and a delightful lathering experience. Formulated with thoughtfully chosen ingredients, it elevates the daily ritual of hair cleansing to a sensory delight.

Key Features:

1. Gentle Cleansing Agents:
    - The shampoo harnesses the power of mild, plant-derived surfactants that cleanse without stripping the hair of its natural oils. This ensures a thorough yet gentle wash.

2. Natural Extracts for Nourishment:
    - Infused with botanical extracts like chamomile and aloe vera, the shampoo nourishes the hair while promoting a soothing and refreshing experience.

3. Aromatic Essential Oils:
    - A carefully curated blend of essential oils, such as lavender

and peppermint, adds not only to the fragrance but also contributes to a calming and invigorating effect during the wash.

4. Sulfate-Free Formula:

   o Free from harsh sulfates, the shampoo ensures a foaming experience without compromising on hair health. It is suitable for a variety of hair types, including color-treated hair.

The Foaming Ritual:

The journey begins with a small amount of the foaming shampoo in the palm of my hand. As I massage it into my wet hair, the luscious foam builds effortlessly, enveloping each strand. The indulgent lather glides smoothly, creating a luxurious experience that extends beyond mere cleansing.

Sensory Pleasure:

The aroma of essential oils fills the air, creating a mini aromatherapy session. The calming lavender intertwines with the invigorating notes of peppermint, turning the shower into a haven of relaxation.

Post-Wash Bliss:

Rinsing is a breeze, leaving my hair feeling clean, soft, and delicately scented. The absence of residue ensures that my hair maintains its natural bounce and vitality.

A Sustainable Touch:

Packaged in an eco-friendly container, my favorite foaming shampoo aligns with a commitment to sustainability. It reflects an awareness that self-care can extend beyond

personal benefits to embrace the well-being of
the planet.

Conclusion:

A favorite foaming shampoo is more than a
hair care product; it's a sensorial journey that
turns a routine task into a cherished ritual.
From the careful selection of ingredients to the
soothing lather and lingering fragrance, each
element contributes to an experience that
transforms a simple wash into a moment of
self-indulgence and well-deserved pampering.

Natural hair conditioners

Nourishing Locks: The Magic of Natural Hair Conditioners

Introduction:

In the realm of hair care, the embrace of natural ingredients extends beyond cleansing to the enriching realm of conditioners. Natural hair conditioners, crafted from botanical treasures, offer a holistic approach to nurturing and revitalizing strands, leaving behind a touch of nature's magic.

Key Ingredients and Their Benefits:

1. Coconut Oil:

    - Renowned for its moisturizing properties, coconut oil penetrates hair strands, providing deep hydration and combating frizz.

2. Shea Butter:

      o Extracted from the shea tree,
         shea butter is a natural emollient
         that seals in moisture, promotes
         elasticity, and enhances hair
         texture.

3. Aloe Vera Gel:

      o Aloe vera soothes the scalp,
         reduces irritation, and contributes
         to overall hair health with its
         hydrating and healing properties.

4. Honey:

      o With its humectant properties,
         honey attracts and retains
         moisture, making it an excellent
         natural conditioner for dry or
         damaged hair.

5. Jojoba Oil:

- Similar to the natural oils
    produced by the scalp, jojoba oil
    adds shine, softens hair, and aids
    in detangling.

DIY Natural Hair Conditioner Recipe:

Ingredients:

- 2 tablespoons coconut oil
- 1 tablespoon shea butter
- 1 tablespoon aloe vera gel
- 1 tablespoon honey
- 1 tablespoon jojoba oil

Instructions:

1. Melt the Shea Butter:

- Shea butter should be melted into a liquid in a double boiler.

2. Combine Ingredients:

   - Mix the melted shea butter with coconut oil, aloe vera gel, honey, and jojoba oil in a bowl. Stir until well combined.

3. Application:

   - Concentrating on the lengths and ends of the hair, apply the mixture to moist, clean hair. To properly distribute the conditioner, use a wide-tooth comb.

4. Wrap and Wait:

   - Cover your hair with a shower cap or towel and leave the conditioner on for at least 30

minutes to allow the ingredients
to penetrate the hair.

5. Rinse Thoroughly:

    o Rinse your hair thoroughly with
       lukewarm water. Style as usual.

Benefits of Natural Hair Conditioners:

1. Hydration and Moisture:

    o Natural conditioners deeply
       moisturize, preventing dryness
       and promoting softer, more
       manageable hair.

2. Improved Hair Texture:

    o Regular use enhances hair
       texture, making it smoother,
       shinier, and less prone to
       breakage.

3. Scalp Health:

- Ingredients like aloe vera contribute to a healthier scalp, reducing irritation and supporting overall hair well-being.

4. Chemical-Free:
    - Free from harsh chemicals, natural conditioners are gentle on both your hair and the environment.

Conclusion:

Natural hair conditioners go beyond cosmetic enhancements; they are a celebration of the earth's nurturing offerings. From coconut oil's tropical embrace to aloe vera's soothing touch, these conditioners embody the essence of holistic hair care, leaving you with tresses that radiate health and vitality.

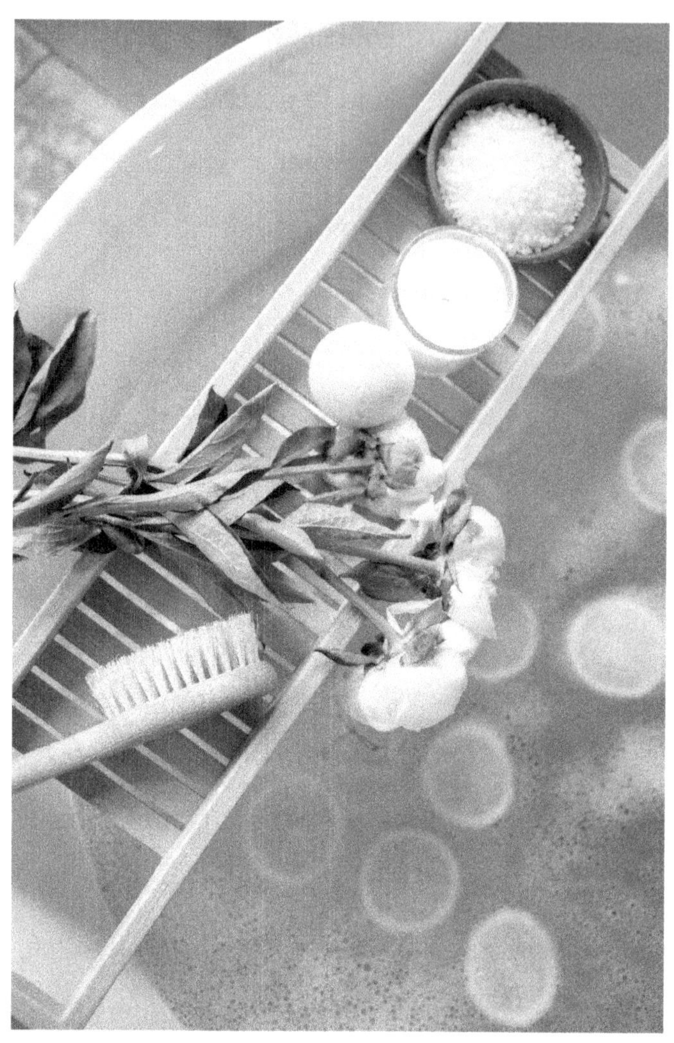

Chapter seven

Herbs and spices

Herbs and Spices: Nature's Culinary and Medicinal Treasures

Introduction:

Herbs and spices, revered for their aromatic flavors and medicinal properties, have been integral to human culture for centuries. These culinary and botanical wonders not only enhance the taste of our dishes but also contribute to a tapestry of holistic health and well-being.

Culinary Magic:

1. Basil:

    ○ This fragrant herb adds a fresh, slightly peppery flavor to dishes, making it a staple in Mediterranean cuisine.

2. Cinnamon:
   - Known for its warm and sweet taste, cinnamon elevates both sweet and savory dishes, imparting a comforting aroma.

3. Rosemary:
   - With a pine-like fragrance, rosemary complements roasted meats and vegetables, adding a robust and earthy flavor.

4. Turmeric:
   - A golden-hued spice, turmeric not only imparts a warm, bitter taste but also contains curcumin, known for its anti-inflammatory properties.

5. Cilantro:

○ Fresh and citrusy, cilantro is a versatile herb used in various cuisines, adding brightness to salads, salsas, and curries.

Medicinal Marvels:

1. Ginger:

    ○ A remedy for digestive discomfort, ginger also possesses anti-inflammatory properties and is commonly used to alleviate nausea.

2. Garlic:

    ○ Beyond its culinary uses, garlic has antimicrobial properties and is believed to support heart health and immune function.

3. Peppermint:

- Known for its soothing properties, peppermint can ease indigestion and alleviate headaches. It's also commonly used in teas.

4. Chamomile:

   - Recognized for its calming effects, chamomile is often brewed into a tea to promote relaxation and aid in sleep.

5. Cayenne Pepper:

   - The compound capsaicin in cayenne pepper not only adds heat to dishes but also has been studied for its potential pain-relieving properties.

Culinary and Wellness Fusion:

1. Turmeric Latte:

- Create a soothing turmeric latte by blending turmeric with warm milk, honey, and a dash of cinnamon for a comforting and healthful beverage.

2. Herb-Infused Oils:

   - Craft your own herb-infused oils using rosemary, thyme, or basil to elevate the flavor of salads or roasted vegetables.

3. Ginger Lemon Tea:

   - Brew a revitalizing ginger lemon tea by steeping fresh ginger and a slice of lemon in hot water for a refreshing beverage.

4. Cilantro Lime Dressing:

   - Blend cilantro, lime juice, garlic, and olive oil to create a zesty dressing for salads or grilled dishes.

Conclusion:

Herbs and spices weave a rich tapestry of flavors in our culinary experiences while offering an array of potential health benefits. As we explore the vast world of these botanical wonders, we not only embark on a journey of taste but also embrace the wisdom of traditional medicine and the innate connection between nature and nourishment.

Chapter eight

Natural Hair Gel

DIY Natural Hair Gel Recipes:

Nourishing Your Tresses with Nature's Goodness

Creating your own natural hair gel allows you to tailor the formula to your hair's specific needs while avoiding harsh chemicals commonly found in commercial products. Here are two simple and effective DIY recipes using natural ingredients:

Aloe Vera Flaxseed Hair Gel:

Ingredients:

- 1/4 cup flaxseeds
- 2 cups water

- 2 tablespoons aloe vera gel

Instructions:

1. Boil Flaxseeds:
   - In a small saucepan, boil flaxseeds in water until it forms a gel-like consistency. Stir occasionally.
2. Strain and Cool:
   - Once the mixture thickens, strain out the flaxseeds, and let the gel cool to room temperature.
3. Add Aloe Vera:
   - Mix in aloe vera gel with the flaxseed gel and stir until well combined.
4. Storage:

- After transferring the gel into a sanitized container, keep it chilled. It will last for approximately two weeks.

Usage:

- Apply a small amount to damp or dry hair for styling or defining curls.

Coconut Lavender Hair Gel:

Ingredients:

- 1/2 cup coconut oil
- 1 teaspoon aloe vera gel
- 10 drops lavender essential oil

Instructions:

1. Blend Ingredients:

    - In a blender, combine coconut oil, aloe vera gel, and lavender essential oil. Blend until a smooth consistency is achieved.

2. Refrigerate:

    - Place the mixture in the refrigerator for about 30 minutes to let it solidify slightly.

3. Whip the Gel:

    - Once slightly solidified, whip the mixture using a hand mixer until it becomes a creamy, gel-like texture.

4. Storage:

    - Transfer the gel into a jar and store it in a cool place.

Usage:

- Take a small amount and rub it between your palms before applying it to your hair for styling or taming frizz.

Tips:

- Experiment with essential oils like peppermint, tea tree, or rosemary for added benefits and a personalized fragrance.
- Adjust the quantities of ingredients based on your hair type and desired consistency.
- Before taking any new product, run a patch test to make sure you don't experience any negative side effects.

These DIY natural hair gels offer a blend of nourishing ingredients, giving your hair a healthy and natural hold without the unwanted chemicals found in many commercial options.

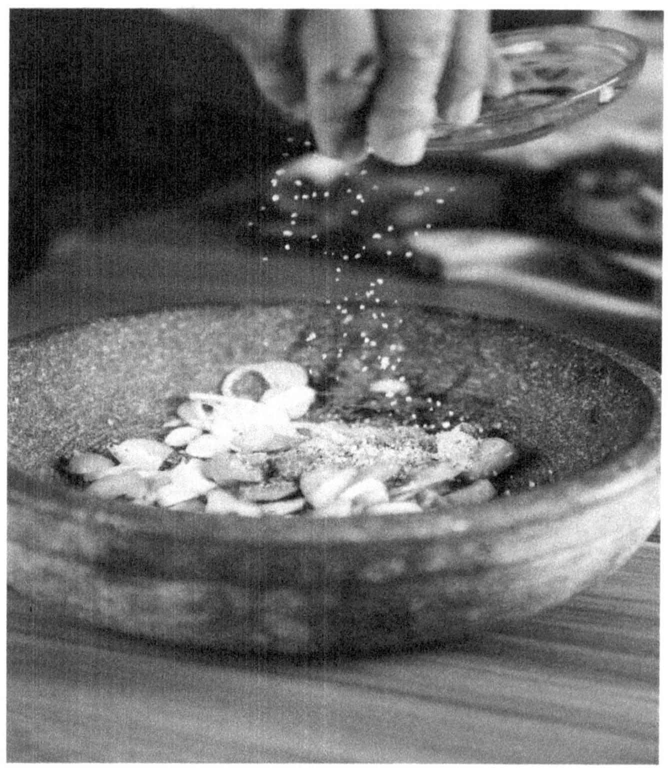

Chapter nine

Healthy hair with a great hair Rinse

Nourishing Elegance: Creating a Healthy Hair Rinse for Lustrous Locks

A homemade hair rinse is a delightful way to infuse your hair care routine with natural ingredients that promote health and shine. Here's a rejuvenating recipe for a hair rinse that will leave your locks looking and feeling fabulous:

Herbal Infusion Hair Rinse:

Ingredients:

- 2 tablespoons dried rosemary
- 2 tablespoons dried chamomile flowers
- 1 tablespoon apple cider vinegar

- 2 cups hot water

Instructions:

1. Create the Herbal Infusion:
   - In a heatproof bowl, combine dried rosemary and chamomile flowers. Cover all of the herbs with a layer of boiling water. Let it steep for at least 30 minutes to allow the herbs to infuse.
2. Strain the Infusion:
   - After steeping, strain the herbal infusion to remove the plant material. Ensure you have a clear liquid.
3. Add Apple Cider Vinegar:
   - Mix apple cider vinegar into the herbal infusion. This provides a

balancing effect and adds shine to your hair.

4. Cool to Room Temperature:
   - Allow the mixture to cool to room temperature. Putting it in the refrigerator can expedite the process.

5. Usage:
   - Use the herbal infusion as a last-minute rinse on your hair after washing.
   - Ensure it covers your hair from root to tip.

6. Do Not Rinse Out:
   - Let the herbal infusion remain in your hair; there's no need to rinse it out. Style your hair as usual.

Benefits of Herbal Hair Rinse:

1. Scalp Health:

    - Rosemary is known for promoting a healthy scalp, reducing dandruff, and encouraging hair growth.

2. Shine Enhancement:

    - Chamomile adds a natural sheen to the hair, leaving it looking glossy and radiant.

3. Balancing pH:

    - Apple cider vinegar helps balance the pH of your hair, promoting a healthy environment for the scalp and hair strands.

4. Aromatic Pleasure:

    - The infusion of rosemary and chamomile provides a delightful and calming fragrance, turning

your hair care routine into a
spa-like experience.

Tips:

- Adjust the quantities of herbs based on your hair length and personal preferences.
- For an extra boost, consider adding a few drops of essential oils such as lavender or tea tree to the rinse.

Incorporating this herbal infusion hair rinse into your routine offers a refreshing and natural way to maintain healthy, lustrous hair. Enjoy the soothing benefits of botanicals while elevating the overall health and beauty of your locks.

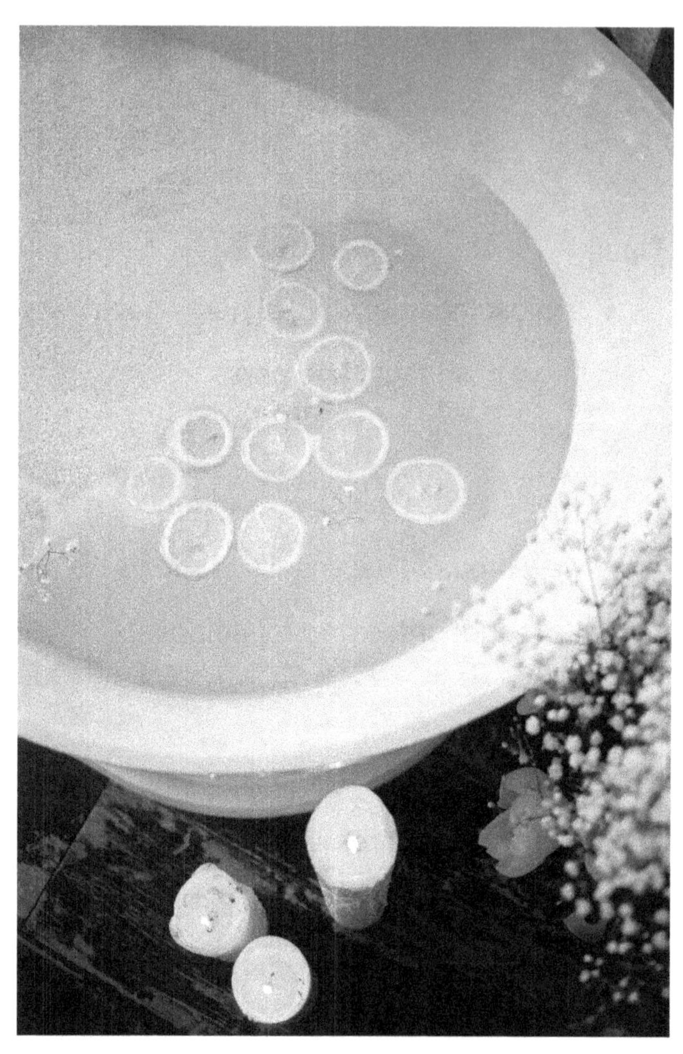

Chapter ten

The Best Recipes to Style Hair

DIY Natural Hair Styling Recipes for Effortless Elegance

Creating your own natural hair styling products allows you to tailor formulations to your hair's unique needs while avoiding harmful chemicals. Here are two versatile recipes for styling hair with natural ingredients:

1. Flaxseed Gel for Defined Curls:

Ingredients:

- 1/4 cup flaxseeds
- 2 cups water
- 1 tablespoon aloe vera gel

- 5-10 drops of your favorite essential oil (e.g., lavender or peppermint)

Instructions:

1. Boil Flaxseeds:
   - In a small saucepan, boil flaxseeds in water until it forms a gel-like consistency. Stir occasionally.
2. Strain and Cool:
   - Once the mixture thickens, strain out the flaxseeds, and let the gel cool to room temperature.
3. Add Aloe Vera and Essential Oil:
   - Mix in aloe vera gel and essential oil with the flaxseed gel. Stir until well combined.
4. Storage:

- After transferring the gel into a sanitized container, keep it chilled. It will last for approximately two weeks.

Usage:

- Apply a small amount to damp or dry hair for styling or defining curls.

2. Coconut Oil Hair Wax for Textured Looks:

Ingredients:

- 1/2 cup coconut oil
- 2 tablespoons beeswax pellets
- 10 drops of your preferred essential oil (e.g., cedarwood or bergamot)

Instructions:

1. Melt Coconut Oil and Beeswax:
   - In a double boiler, melt coconut oil and beeswax pellets together. Stir until well combined.
2. Cool Slightly:
   - Allow the mixture to cool slightly but not solidify completely.
3. Add Essential Oil:
   - Stir in your chosen essential oil for fragrance and additional benefits.
4. Storage:
   - Pour the mixture into a container and let it solidify completely. Store in a cool, dry place.

Usage:

- To warm it up, take a little bit and massage it between your hands. Apply to dry hair for a textured, controlled look.

Tips:

- Adjust the quantity of essential oil based on your preferred fragrance intensity.
- Experiment with different essential oils to customize the scent and add unique benefits.
- Store these products in airtight containers to prolong their shelf life.

These DIY natural styling products offer a healthy alternative to commercial hair styling products, providing nourishment and hold without the use of harsh chemicals. Enjoy the versatility and benefits of these natural recipes for effortlessly styled and beautifully maintained hair.

Ultimate guide to Avoiding hair loss

The Ultimate Guide to Preventing Hair Loss Naturally

Hair loss can be a distressing concern, but adopting a holistic approach to your hair care routine and overall health can contribute to preventing and minimizing hair loss. Here's a comprehensive guide to help you maintain a healthy head of hair:

1. Nutrient-Rich Diet:

- Key Nutrients: Ensure your diet includes a balance of essential nutrients like

vitamins A, C, D, and E, as well as
minerals such as iron, zinc, and biotin,
which play crucial roles in hair health.

2. Scalp Care:
- Regular Cleansing: Keep your scalp
  clean to prevent clogged hair follicles,
  but avoid excessive washing, which can
  strip the scalp of natural oils.
- Massage: Stimulate blood flow to the
  scalp through gentle massages to
  promote nutrient delivery to the hair
  follicles.

3. Gentle Hair Care:
- Avoid Harsh Chemicals: Limit the use of
  chemical-laden hair products and
  choose sulfate-free shampoos and
  conditioners.

- Minimize Heat Styling: Reduce the frequency of heat styling to prevent damage. Use a heat protectant while employing heat.

4. **Natural Hair Masks:

- Egg Mask: Mix an egg with olive oil and apply as a mask for protein and moisture.
- Aloe Vera Mask: Aloe vera promotes scalp health and can be applied as a mask or in combination with other nourishing ingredients.

5. **Manage Stress:

- Relaxation Techniques: Practice stress-management techniques such as meditation, yoga, or deep breathing exercises.

- Adequate Sleep: Ensure you get enough quality sleep as lack of sleep can contribute to hair loss.

6. Stay Hydrated:

- Water Intake: Hydrate your body by drinking enough water to support overall health, including hair health.

7. Regular Exercise:

- Cardiovascular Activities: Engage in regular exercise to improve blood circulation, delivering essential nutrients to the hair follicles.

8. Avoid Tight Hairstyles:

- Loose Styles: Choose hairstyles that don't pull on the hair follicles, avoiding tight braids or ponytails.

9. **Protect Hair from UV Rays:

- Hats or Scarves: Shield your hair from the sun's damaging UV rays by wearing hats or scarves.

10. **Consult a Professional:

- Dermatologist or Trichologist: If you experience persistent or severe hair loss, consult with a dermatologist or trichologist for personalized advice.

11. **Consider Supplements:

- Consult a Healthcare Professional: Discuss with a healthcare professional the potential benefits of supplements like biotin, omega-3 fatty acids, or other hair-friendly nutrients.

12. **Avoid Smoking:

- Quit Smoking: Smoking can contribute to hair loss, so quitting can improve overall health, including the health of your hair.

Conclusion:

Preventing hair loss involves adopting a holistic approach that considers your overall health, lifestyle, and hair care practices. By nourishing your body and hair, managing stress, and adopting a gentle hair care routine, you can promote a healthy scalp and maintain a vibrant head of hair. If concerns persist, seeking professional advice ensures tailored guidance for your specific situation.

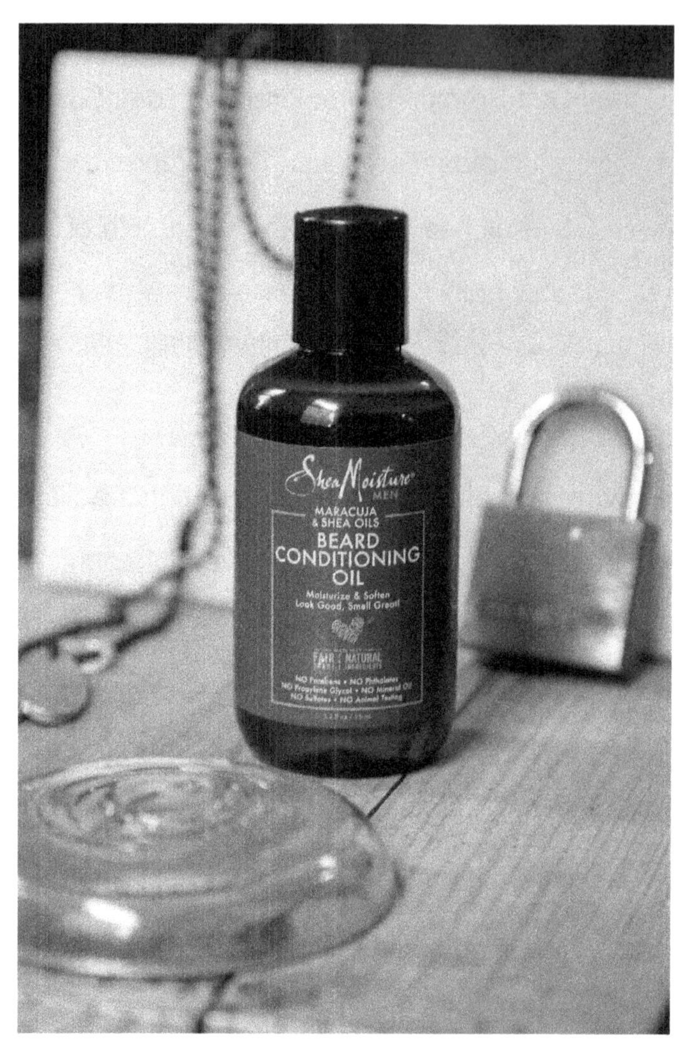
SheaMoisture
MEN
MARACUJA
& SHEA OILS
BEARD
CONDITIONING
OIL
Moisturize & Soften
Look Good, Smell Great!
FAIR NATURAL

Conclusion

In conclusion, natural hair care recipes offer a harmonious blend of nature's bounty and holistic well-being for your tresses. From nourishing hair masks to revitalizing rinses and styling products crafted from herbs, essential oils, and kitchen staples, these recipes provide a wholesome alternative to commercial products laden with chemicals. Embracing the nutrient-rich goodness of ingredients like coconut oil, aloe vera, and essential oils not only enhances the health of your hair but also creates a sensorial experience that transforms routine care into a moment of self-indulgence.

The versatility of natural hair care recipes shines through, addressing a spectrum of needs from deep conditioning and styling to promoting scalp health and preventing hair loss. Whether you're seeking luscious curls, textured looks, or simply a radiant mane, these DIY recipes allow for customization, catering to your unique hair type and preferences.

Furthermore, the emphasis on mindful practices, such as scalp massages, gentle hair care routines, and stress management, underscores the holistic nature of natural hair care. By adopting these recipes, you not only nourish your hair but also cultivate a connection to nature's wonders, fostering a healthier and more sustainable approach to self-care.

As you embark on this journey of natural hair care, experimenting with different recipes and discovering what works best for you adds an element of joy to your daily routine. The beauty of natural hair care lies not just in the outcomes

– soft, shiny, and well-styled hair – but in the process itself, where each application becomes a ritual, a celebration of the wholesome goodness that nature provides.

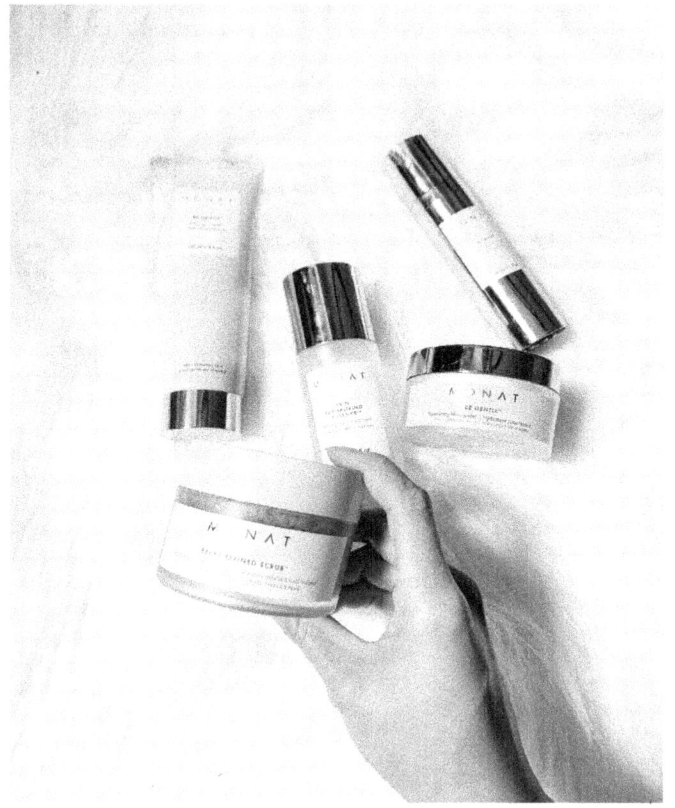